Elf-help
for Coping
with Pain

Elf-help for Coping with Pain

written by
Anne Calodich Fone

illustrated by
R.W. Alley

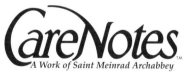

CareNotes™
A Work of Saint Meinrad Archabbey

Saint Meinrad Archabbey
200 Hill Drive
St. Meinrad, IN 47577
ElfHelpbooks.com • CareNotes.com

Text © 2019 by Anne Calodich Fone
Illustrations © 2019 by Saint Meinrad Archabbey
Published by CareNotes
St. Meinrad, Indiana 47577

Library of Congress Catalog Number
2002111018

ISBN 978-0-87029-368-9

Printed in the United States of America.

Foreword

Rarely is life's landscape level. Pain comes uninvited, moving mountains into our paths. Pain brings change and change brings challenge. But mountains can be climbed and challenges can be met.

We are each the work of a loving Creator, a wondrous integration of mind and body, spirit and emotions. When one or more of these parts is out of balance, pain acts as a warning, signaling us to respond.

Elf-help for Coping With Pain offers no quick-fix solutions. What it does offer are gentle reminders that any journey from woundedness to wholeness is a process and not meant to be traveled alone. There are things you can do to make the trip easier. There are blessings to be found along the way.

Whether the pain with which you are coping is short-term or chronic, injury or illness, trauma or loss, you will find within these pages both words and illustrations that will encourage and inspire.

May the following suggestions for finding resources and strength within God, yourself, and others help motivate you to face your future with faith and with hope.

1.

In our lives, pain is inevitable. In His love, God is indomitable. Allow your mind and your spirit to accept both of these truths.

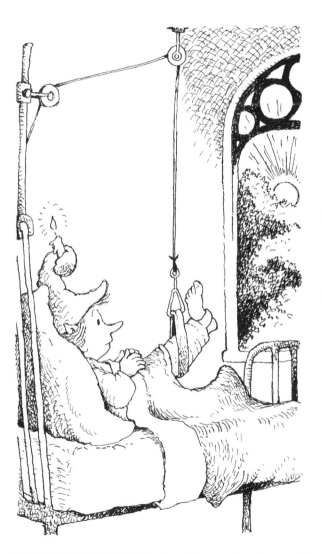

2.

You cannot possess what you cannot perceive. "You are what you think you are." Develop a mentality that survives rather than merely endures, conquers rather than merely lives wounded.

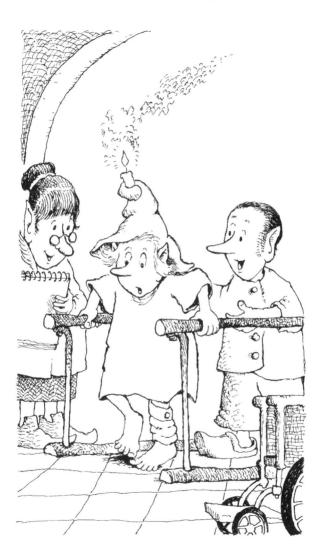

3.

Become your own advocate
by searching out information.
Read, ask questions, research
the internet, contact
professionals and/or those
in similar situations to your
own. From this well-informed
stance, you will be in a better
position to assess your options
and set realistic goals.

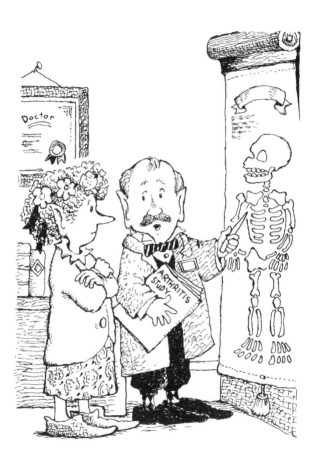

4.

Although you may have
to accept some short-term
restrictions at present, reject
any long-term limitations as
permanent. Both time and
perspective will teach you
new ways to adjust and adapt.

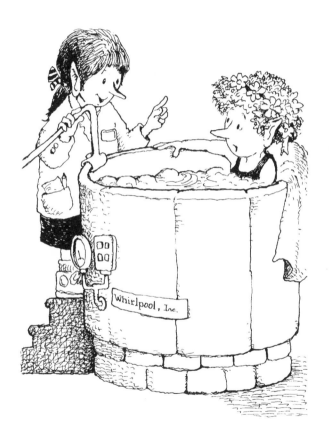

5.

Anxiety, fear, and depression can actually add to pain's intensity. Dare to share. Hearing your own feelings spoken aloud to a trusted friend, family member, spiritual or professional counselor can help to clear the fog and make them easier to confront.

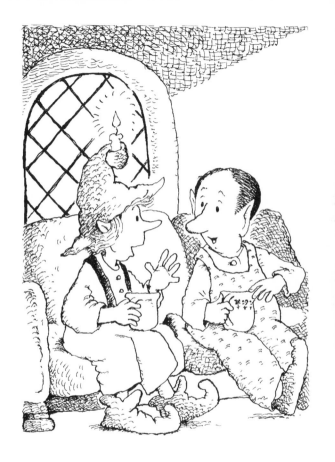

6.

Pain can teach us how to prioritize. You may now see new purpose and value in what you passed by in busyness before. Do some mental math: What can you add to your life to make it more meaningful? What can you subtract?

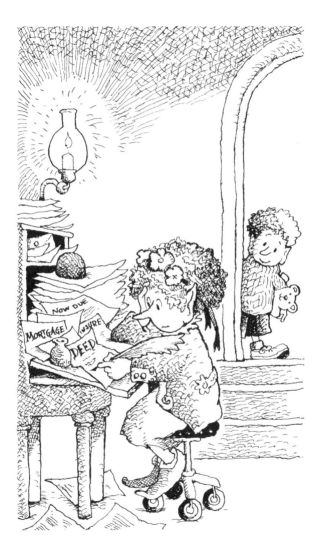

7.

Check your life for balance. Routine leaves us rigid and restless in our own self-made ruts. Make sure your "TO DO" list includes activities you know or think you'd enjoy as well as obligations that need to be met.

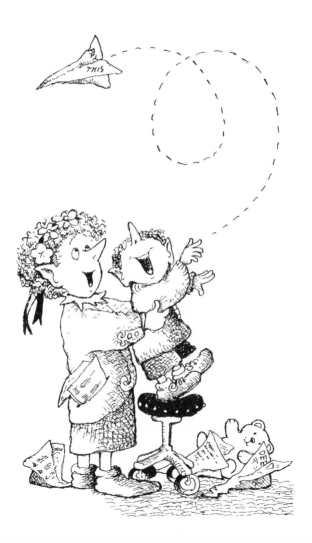

8.

Refuse to give pain the loudest voice. Still your mind and your heart to hear God's guiding whispers. Climb up and cuddle like a child upon your Father's lap as you read God's Word, meditate on God's promises, and carry each concern to God in trustful prayer.

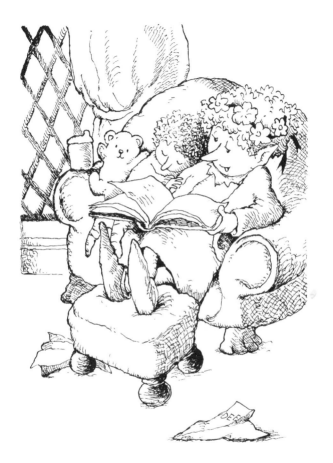

9.

Do not try to bear the whole burden alone. False independence can be self-defeating. True strength is admitting you can't handle it all. Ask for help or for hugs whenever you need them.

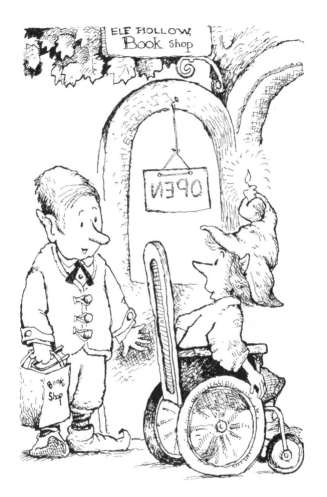

10.

Take responsibility for any part you may have played in your pain. Guilt keeps us looking backward—away from solutions that may lie ahead. Change what you can as you face forward again.

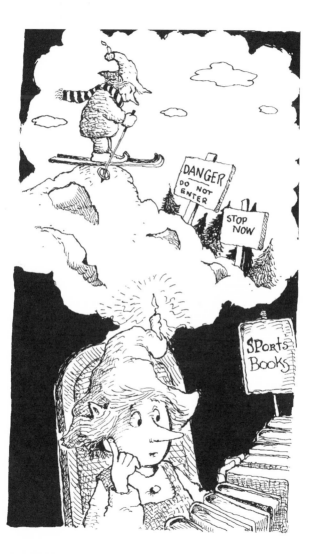

11.

Give yourself the gifts of time, gentleness, and patience. Take time-outs when feeling frustrated or discouraged. Deep breaths, calming thoughts, and forgiveness of self and of others can do wonders to putting yourself back on track.

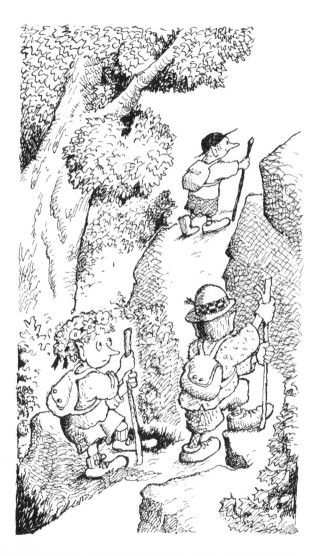

12.

Resist the temptation to compare yourself to others. There is a world of difference between "limitation" and "weakness," between "inability" and "unwillingness." Measure your progress only by those steps that you take to meet your own specific goals.

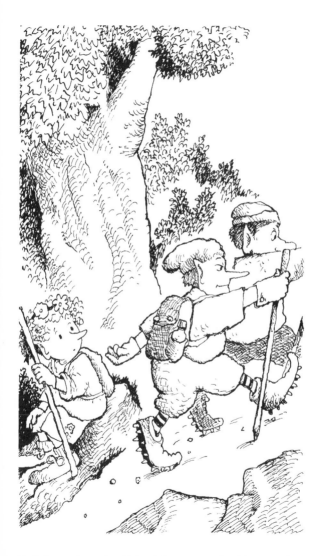

13.

Positive self-talk can help bring about healing. Become your own cheerleader as you applaud each of your efforts. Remind yourself daily that each step you attempt is a potential victory, giving voice to the fact that you have not, that you will not, give up.

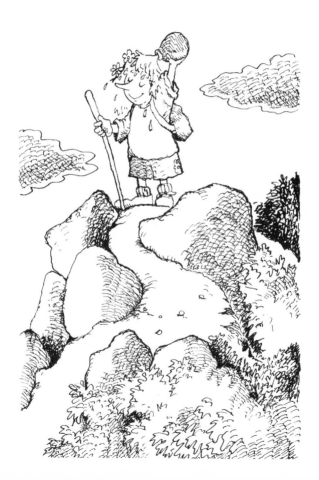

14.

Don't resort to unhealthy habits
in an attempt to dull the pain.
What we choose to do now,
we WILL pay for later.
Become your own watchdog
as you guard against those
choices that will more likely
harm than help.

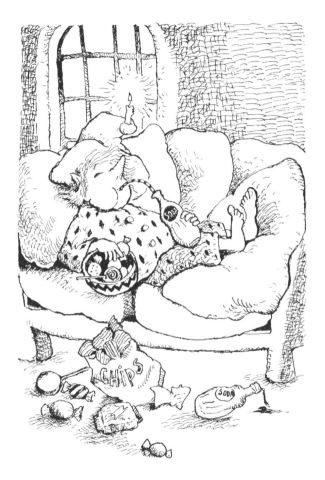

15.

Keep your eyes completely on God as you grieve any losses. Carry your cares to the One who never stops caring. Converse with God honestly about all your emotions.

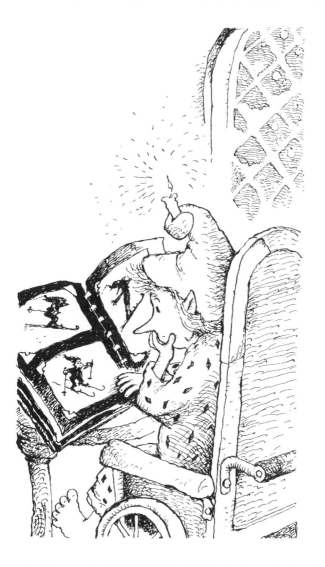

16.

Learn to listen to those messages your mind and body may be sending. Respond gently with gifts like sunlight, rest, meditation, and nature; respond firmly with disciplines like exercise, study, good nutrition, and work. Feel yourself returning to your own natural balance.

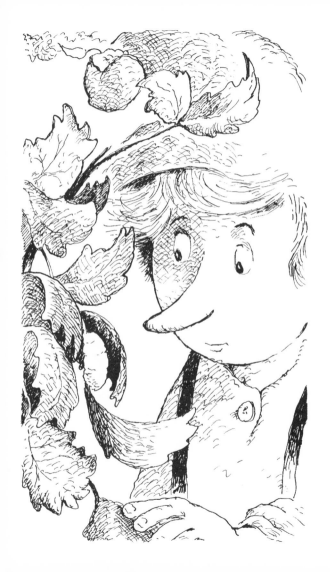

17.

Savor the miracle held in each moment. If you allow it, pain can heighten your senses, revealing more of life's beauty: the intricacy of a flower, the sunlight dancing on the wall, a memory as it brushes your cheek. Examine, experience, enjoy!

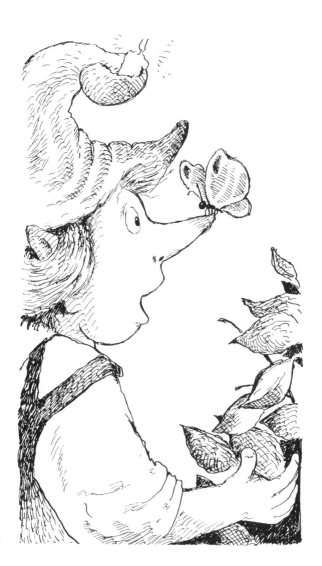

18.

Just as crying, at times, can cleanse you of pain, humor can help anesthetize you to it. Make it a habit to surround yourself with people who tickle your funny bone. Choose videos or television programs that make you laugh right out loud.

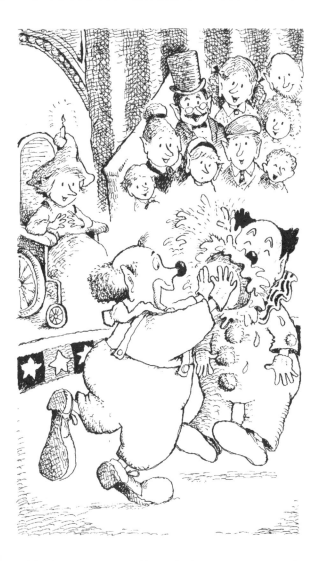

19.

Consider visiting a nutritionist. Unhealthy bodies, minds, and resulting emotions can often be traced back to poor diet, food allergies, and vitamin or mineral deficiencies. A nutritionist can also guide you through the maze of natural and herbal remedies while teaching you how to make healthy choices.

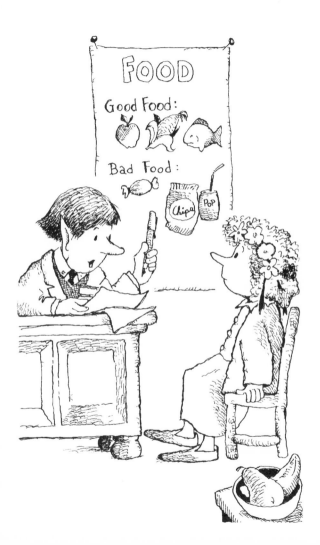

20.

Commit to follow through on all you plan to do. Giving up too easily or early can sabotage your efforts to alleviate your pain. Give each choice enough time to produce honest results.

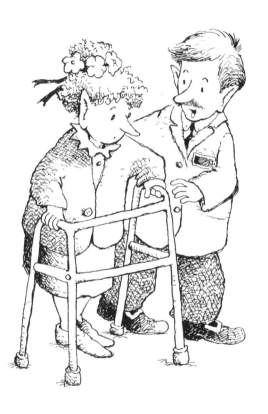

21.

At times, you may feel no one understands. When this happens, resist the urge to disconnect from people. After all, we have all experienced pain to some degree, and empathy is one of God's strongest reminders that we are in so many ways similar.

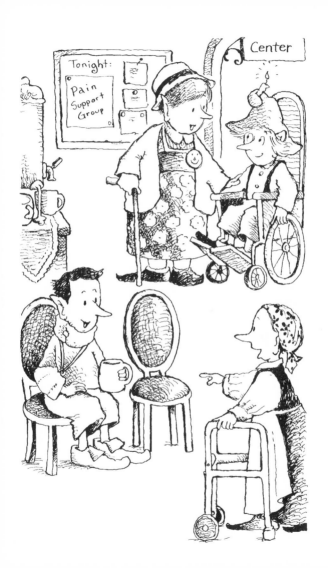

22.

Use imagination to help you break through pain's boundaries. Try your creative hand at such pursuits as painting, writing, photography, or music. If not your own, simply enjoy the vast array of contributions others have made to such fields.

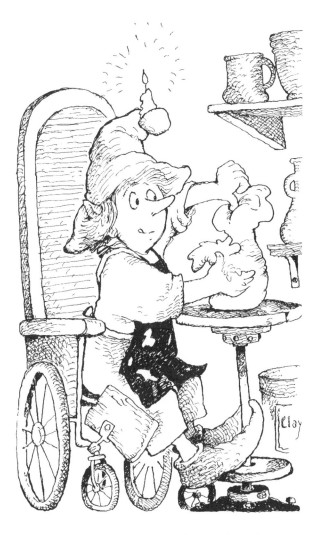

23.

Color your days with thanksgiving and praise! Step outside of yourself and your pain to acknowledge all that God is and has given to us. Feel God's peace and love lift you above the cares and concerns of this world.

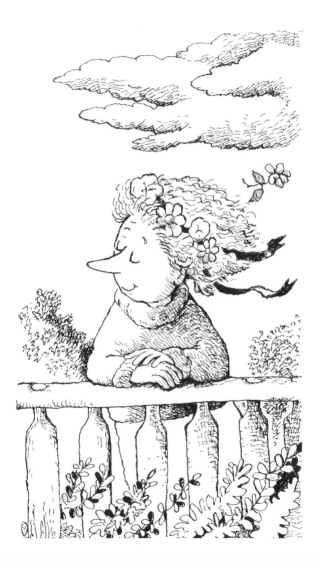

24.

Think about getting a pet. Studies show tending to and nurturing an animal, while receiving its unconditional love, can help lower blood pressure, renew a sense of purpose, and brighten your outlook.

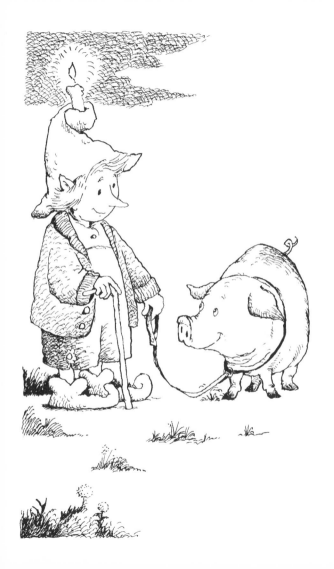

25.

Create a Faith Box. Into an attractive container, place all those scriptures, quotes, inspirational cards and messages that cause your spirit to soar. Open as needed.

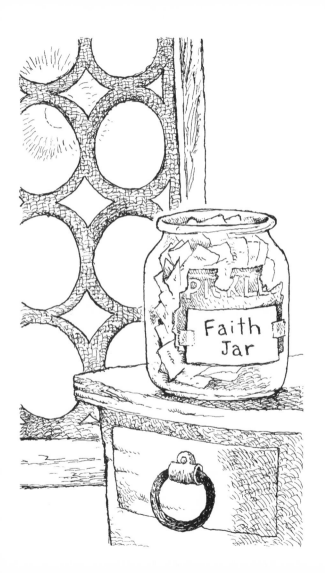

26.

Stop replaying the past.
Make peace with anyone with
whom you have differences.
Forgiveness can release those
toxins of anger, resentment,
and bitterness that may be
blocking your healing.

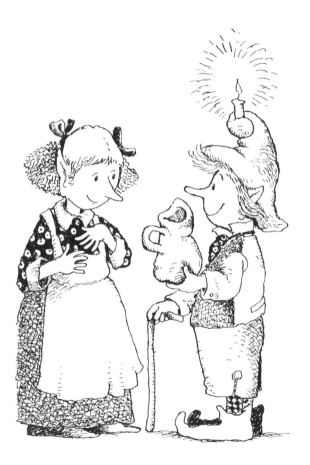

27.

The more your mind and body relax, the more pain and stress have an opportunity to lessen. Explore such possibilities as deep breathing exercises, aromatherapy, daily prayer and meditation, herbal baths, progressive muscle relaxation, and therapeutic massage. Discover which work best for you.

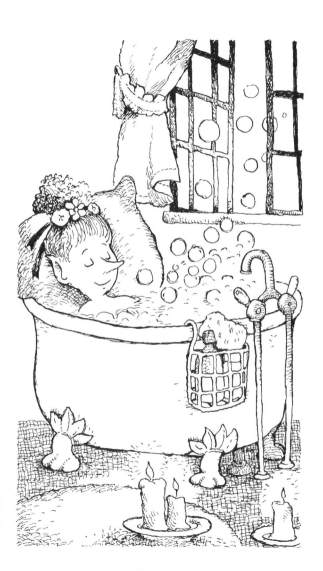

28.

Recognize the wisdom, resolve,
and new growth being forged
in the heart of your pain.
Experience is one of our greatest
instructors. Record in a journal
the insights you have gained
and the gifts being received
throughout this journey.

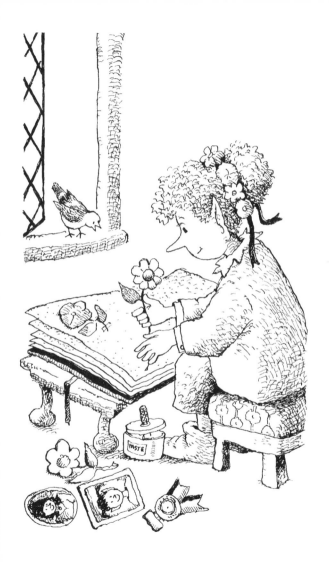

29.

An absence of pain would leave us with an absence of compassion. Be a blessing! Comfort as you have been comforted. No matter how you may feel, you can still encourage another with a word, with a prayer, with a smile, with your care.

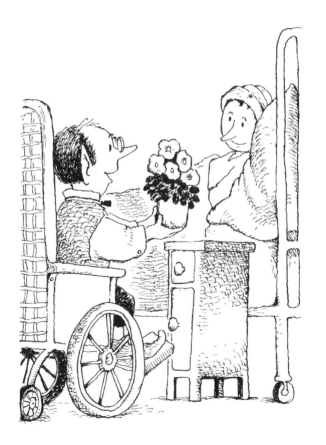

30.

Everything feels worse when you're tired. Aim for at least eight hours a night by maintaining a regular sleep routine. If you have had a bad night, try to re-schedule your day to include breaks or naps.

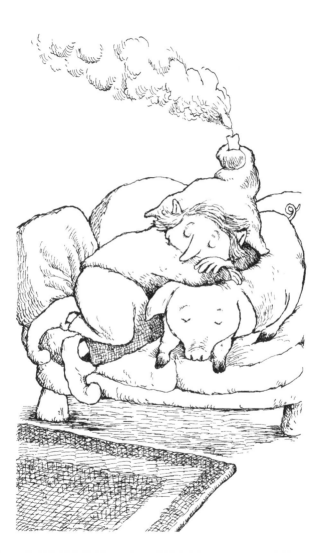

31.

Make your environment as pleasant as possible. De-cluttering a room can help de-clutter the mind, leaving you feeling more in control. Surrounding yourself with soothing colors, favorite fabrics, and personal treasures can help elevate your mood and keep your heart smiling.

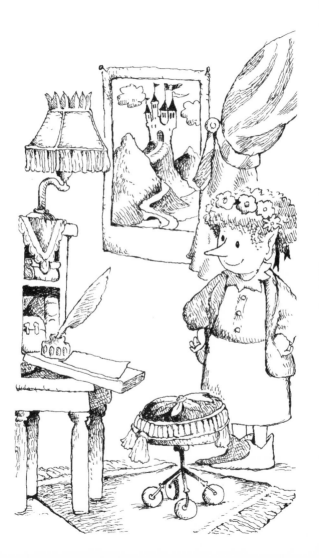

32.

Keep a pain diary. Tracking its ebbs and its flows, as well as pinpointing any particular triggers, can help you and those working with you formulate a more personal pain-management plan.

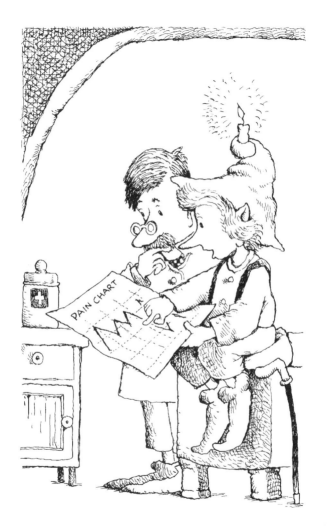

33.

Figure out brand new ways to make old dreams come true. Though pain may slow you down, it does not have to place you outside of the race. Pursue...Persist...Persevere.

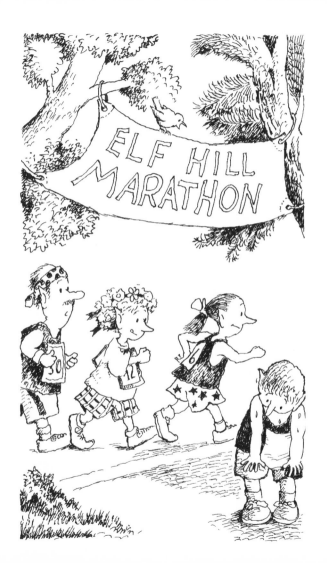

34.

Fear exaggerates life's worst while faith exemplifies God's best. Remembering how faithful God has been in your yesterdays can help ease the pain of today.

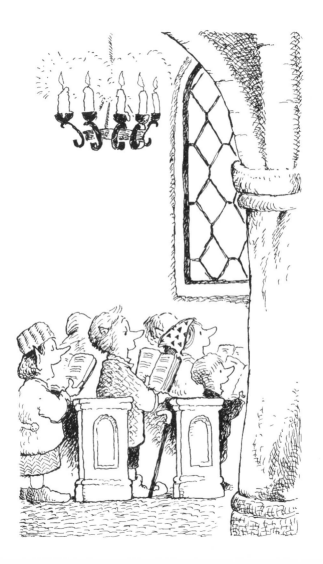

35.

Remember, the gift of true joy is always heart-near. Wrap yourself in the warmth of all the love you are wished. Cozy yourself in the comfort of all who truly care.

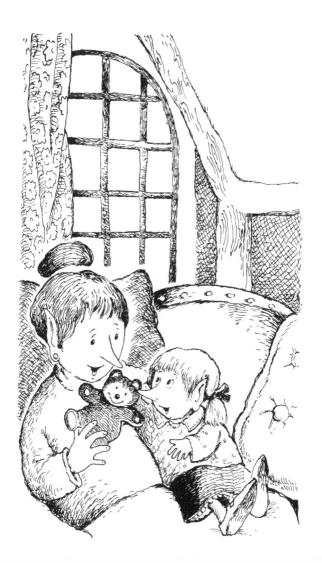

36.

Although God is not the author of your pain, God remains present with you in it. When you feel yourself getting lost in confusion, find peace in remembering God still has purpose for your life.

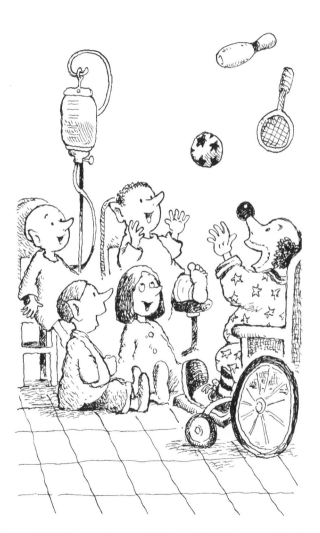

37.

Look for those new paths to which your pain may point you. A change in direction can propel you to undreamed-of possibilities. A simple detour can provide the adventure of a lifetime!

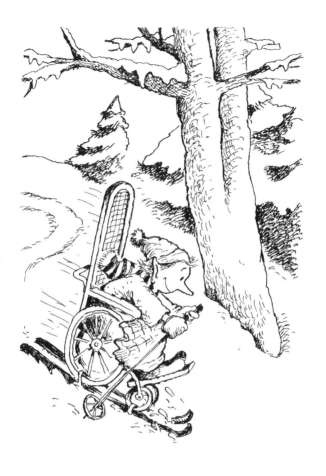

38.

When pain brings us to the end of ourselves, we come to the beginning of God. It is within our weakness that we find God's grace sufficient. Hold on to this grace as you surrender your final healing to God.

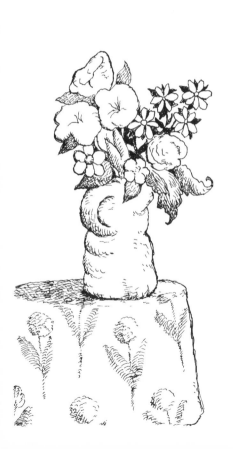

Anne Calodich Fone is a former elementary and special education teacher who has worked with the physically, mentally, and emotionally challenged. She believes it is her own experiences with chronic pain which led her to change careers and begin a ministry of encouragement through her writing. Originally from Brooklyn, Anne and her husband, Larry, have raised a daughter, Katie, and now live in upstate New York.

Illustrator for the Saint Meinrad Archabbey Elf-help Books, **R.W. Alley** also illustrates and writes children's books. He lives in Barrington, Rhode Island, with his wife, daughter, and son. See a wide variety of his works at: www.rwalley.com.

The Story of the Elves

The engaging figures that populate the Saint Meinrad Archabbey "elf-help" line of publications and products first appeared in 1987 on the pages of a small self-help book called *Be-good-to-yourself Therapy*. Shaped by the publishing staff's vision and defined in R.W. Alley's inventive illustrations, they lived out author Cherry Hartman's gentle, self-nurturing advice with charm, poignancy, and humor.

Reader response was so enthusiastic that more Elf-help Books were soon under way, a still-growing series that has inspired a line of related gift products.

The especially endearing character featured in the early books—sporting a cap with a mood-changing candle in its peak—has since been joined by a spirited female elf with flowers in her hair.

These two exuberant, sensitive, resourceful, kindhearted, lovable sprites, along with their lively elfin community, reveal what's truly important as they offer messages of joy and wonder, playfulness and co-creation, wholeness and serenity, the miracle of life and the mystery of God's love.

With wisdom and whimsy, these little creatures with long noses demonstrate the elf-help way to a rich and fulfilling life.

Elf-help Books

**...adding "a little character" and a lot
of help to self-help reading!**

Available at your favorite gift shop or bookstore—
or directly from CareNotes Publications,
St. Meinrad, IN 47577. Or call 1-800-325-2511.
ElfHelpBooks.com • CareNotes.com